YOUR KNOWLEDGE HAS VALUE

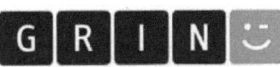

Bibliographic information published by the German National Library:

The German National Library lists this publication in the National Bibliography; detailed bibliographic data are available on the Internet at http://dnb.dnb.de .

Imprint:

Copyright © 2018 GRIN Verlag
Print and binding: Books on Demand GmbH, Norderstedt Germany
ISBN: 9783668700505

This book at GRIN:

https://www.grin.com/document/424758

Sagar Pamu

A Review on Supra Ventricular Tachycardia. An ECG Explanation on Irregular Heart Beats

GRIN Verlag

GRIN - Your knowledge has value

Since its foundation in 1998, GRIN has specialized in publishing academic texts by students, college teachers and other academics as e-book and printed book. The website www.grin.com is an ideal platform for presenting term papers, final papers, scientific essays, dissertations and specialist books.

Visit us on the internet:

http://www.grin.com/

http://www.facebook.com/grincom

http://www.twitter.com/grin_com

A REVIEW ON SUPRAVENTRICULAR TACHYCARDIA

Author:

Sagar Pamu

A REVIEW ON SUPRAVENTRICULAR TACHYCARDIA

List of Contents

Inhalt

Introduction of SVT:

Supra Ventricular Tachycardia refers to rapid rhythm of heart for a reason other than exerscise, high fever and stress. This kind of faster heart beats originates and is sustained in atrial or atrioventricular nodal tissue, and then transmits improper electrical activity from upper part of the heart through the bundle of His and cause rapid ventricular response. They may start either from the atria and atrioventricular node.

The heart beats in a normal healthy individual will be atleast a 100 beats per minute but in SVT there may be a heart beat reaches upto 300 beats per minute. Generally many persons with these tachyarrhythmias have structurally normal hearts [1]. SVT may start and stop quickly, and you may not have symptoms. SVT becomes very complicate when it happens often and lasts for a long time or causes its symptoms.

Epidemiology:

The overall prevalence of SVT is two or three per 1,000 persons in the general pop- ulation. The mean age of occurrence is 45 years and 62% of cases occur in women [2]. SVT occurs in one per 250 to 1,000 infants and children, with Atrio Ventricular Re-entrant Tachycardia (AVRT) accounting for most cases [3].

The incidence of Atrio Ventricular Nodal Re-entrant Tachycardia (AVNRT) in women is twice than in men [4]. It is correlated with lower estrogen levels and higher progesterone levels, and is therefore more common during the luteal phase of the menstrual cycle and less common during pregnancy [5].

Atrial Fibrillation (AF) and Atrial flutter (AFL) are the most common subtypes of SVT, affecting approximately 2 million patients in the United States. Of the remaining subtypes of SVT, Atrioventricular Nodal Reentrant Tachycardia (AVNRT) is the most common, accounting for approximately 60% of cases [6].

The subtypes of Atrioventricular Reentrant Tachycardia (AVRT) and atrial tachycardia account for approximately 30% and 10% of SVT cases, respectively [6].

The incidence of Paroxysmal Supra Ventricular Tachycardia is approximately 1-3 cases per 1000 persons, with a prevalence of 0.2%. Atrial fibrillation is affecting 3 million people in the United States alone, with prevalence of 0.4-1% in the population. It is estimated that atrial fibrillation will affect more than 7.5 million people by 2050 [7].

Causes:

SVT and PSVT generally start from either the atria or atrioventricular node. They are triggered due to one of two different mechanisms: one it is reentry or increased automaticity. This may be induced by premature atrial and other type of fast heart rhythm is ventricular arrhythmias- rapid rythms that start within the ventricle.

Some other triggers include hyperthyroidism and stimulants, including caffeine, drugs use such as cocaine and methamphetamines, surgery, pregnancy, which causes SVT [8].

Paroxysmal SVT is observed not only in healthy individuals. It is also common in patients with previous myocardial infarction, mitral valve prolapse, rheumatic Heart Disease, pericarditis, pneumonia, chronic lung disease, and current alcohol intoxication [8]. Digoxin toxicity also may be associated with paroxysmal SVT [9]. Some other health conditions like Wolff-Parkinson-White syndrome also causes the SVT. However majority of cases has no identifiable triggering factors for SVT.

Signs and Symptoms:

PSVT can cause a number of symptoms, depending on a person's overall health and how fast their heart is beating. Compare to healthy persons, patients with heart problems or any other comorbities experience a higher degree of upset or abash and complications. Some individuals may have no symptoms [10].

Symptoms can come on suddenly and may go away by themselves; they can last for a few minutes or as long as 1-2 days. During Paroxysmal SVT, the faster beat of the heart can make the heart less effective pumping, so that the body tissues may not receive sufficient blood to work normally [10].

Palpitations (the sensation of the heart pounding in the chest) Dizziness, light- headedness, fainting, Shortness of breath, Anxiety, chest pain or tightness are the symptoms experienced when the pulse rate is between 140 and 250 beats per minute [10].

SVT Symptoms and Signs in Infants and Children:

In infants and very young children, symptoms are sometimes difficult to identify. Whatever Paroxysmal SVT may have in the infants those with poor feeding, irritability, perspiration, light color of skin, and who reaches a pulse rate of 200-250 beats per minute [11].

To diagnose supraventricular tachycardia, physician reviews the symptoms, medical history and conduct a physical examination. Electrical activity of heart can be detected with the procedures of Electrocardiogram (ECG), sensors (electrodes) which are attached to the chest and sometimes to limbs. An ECG measures the timing and duration of each electrical phase in the heartbeat. Holter monitor is a portable ECG device; this can be worn for a day or more to record the hearts activity.

Diagnosis:

Event monitor is also a portable ECG device; this is used for the sporadic episodes of SVT [12]. In Echocardiogram, a transducer is placed on the chest; this uses sound waves to produce images of heart's structure, size and motion. Implantable loop recorder detects abnormal heart rhythms and is implanted under the skin in the chest area [12].

TREATMENT:

The treatment goal is to slow down the rate and convert to sinus rhythm by increasing the refractoriness of the AV node or blocking of the AV node. This is accomplished with vagal maneuvers, medications, or cardioversion [13].

The patients with frequent episodes, some studies suggest nondiydropyridine calcium channel blockers or beta blockers. This can correct the conduction across the AV node and decrease the number and duration of episodes. The class I C antiarrhythmics flecainide and propafenone depress conduction across an accessory pathway and suppress episodes in

5

most patients. In patient with atrial tachycardia these medications can be suggested.

The class I A medications quinidine, procainamide, and disopyramide are less commonly used because of their modest effectiveness, and adverse and proarrhythmic effects. The drugs like amiodarone, dofetilide and sotalol which belongs to class III medications are effective in management. These medications can have adverse events, so they should be taken with the reference from cardiologist [14].

Carotid sinus massage may show a gentle pressure on the neck, in which the carotid artery divides into two branches to release some chemicals that can slow the rate of heart.

Vagal maneuvers may be able to stop an episode of SVT by using particular maneuvers that include holding breath and straining, dunking face in ice water, or coughing. This procedure of management shows its affect on the nervous system that controls heartbeat, and it often leads to become slow heart rate of the patient [15].

Cardioversion is the process of delivering shock to the heart by placing patches or paddles on the chest. This current affects the electrical impulses in your heart and can restore a normal heart rhythm.

Catheter ablation is the process of threading one or more catheters through blood vessels to the heart. Catheter tips of the electrodes uses heat or radiofrequency energy or extreme heat to destroy a part of heart tissue and generates an electrical block along the pathway which causes arrhythmia [16].

Risk Factors:

SVT is a common type of arrhythmia in infants and children. Although it occurs in either sex, it tends to occur more often in women, especially in pregnant women.

There are some risk factors which may increase the risk of SVT

- **Age:** In middle aged or older some types of supraventricular are more common.

- **Congenital heart disease:** Born with an abnormal heart during birth may affect your hearts rhythm.

- **Coronary artery disease:** Other heart problems and previous heart surgery: Narrowed coronary arteries, a heart attack, abnormal heart valves, History of heart surgery, congestive heart failure, cardiomyopathy and other damages of heart increase the risk of occuring SVT.

- **Thyroid problems:** Patient with an overactive or underactive thyroid gland can develop the risk of SVT.

- **Drugs and supplements:** Over-the-counter drugs related to cough and cold and some other prescription drugs may lead to an episode of SVT.

- **Nicotine and illegal drug use:** Nicotine and illegal drugs, such as cocaine and ampetamines, may have great intense to affect the heart and trigger an episode of SVT.

- **Physical fatigue**

- **Anxiety or emotional stress**

- **Diabetes:** Risk of developing coronary artery disease and hypertension greatly elevates with uncontrolled diabetes.

- **Obstructive sleep apnea:** Breathing interrupttion during sleep, can increase your risk of developing SVT.

Prevention of SVT:

An episode of SVT can prevent by knowing the triggering factor and the episodes to occur SVT triggering factor should avoid. Keep noting the causative things to identify triggering factor and track the rate of heart, activity and symptoms during the time of SVT episodes [17]. Following are the things to follow to avoid from SVT.

- Increase the physical activity

- Have an heart-healthy diet

- Avoid smoking

- Maintain a healthy weight

- Limit or avoid alcohol

- Reduce stress

- Get the plenty of rest

- OTC medications usage should be with caution, as some drugs contain stimulants that may trigger a faster heartbeat

- Avoid stimulant drugs like as cocaine and methamphetamines

For most people with SVT, moderate amounts of caffeine do not affect an episode. Large amounts of caffeine should avoid.

Complications:

Over time, untreated and frequent episodes of supraventricular tachycardia may depress the heart and lead to heart failure, particularly if the patients have other comorbidities. In extreme cases, an episode of SVT may cause unconsciousness or cardiac arrest.

Life Style Modifications:

Life style modifications like eating healty foods (low in salt, solid fats and rich in fruits, vegetables and whole grains), increasing physical activity, reducing and eventuelly avoiding alcohol intake, quitting smoking, maintaining Ideal Body Weight (IBW), mainitaing normal levels of cholesterol and Blood Pressure (BP), following prescription orders etc helps in improving your health condition [18].

Figure No-01: Life Style Modifications of SVT (Avoid Smoking and Alcoholism)

[Image adapted from http://ddinews.gov.in/health/heavy-drinking-and-smoking-can-age-you-faster-study]

Types of SVT's:

- Atrial Fibrillation (AF)

- Atrial Flutter (AFL)

- Paroxysmal Supraventricular Tachycardia (PSVT)

- Atrio Ventricular Nodal Re-entrant Tachycardia (AVNRT)

- Atrio Ventricular Re-entrant Tachycardia (AVRT)

- Wolff–Parkinson–White syndrome (WPW)

Atrial Fibrillation:

Atrial fibrillation can be described as an extreme faster (400 to 600 atrial beats/min) and abnormal activation of atria. There is an absence or loss of atrial contraction, and supraventricular impulses generates the atrioventricualr(AV) conduction system in variable degrees, resulting in irregular ventricular activation and irregularly irregular pulse (120 to 180 beats/ min) [19].

Atrial fibrillation is a frequent and unexpected cardiac arrhythmia [20]. Atrial fibrillation is an age dependent affecting 4% older than 60 years and 8% older than 80 years. Almost 25% of the SVT patients aged 40 years and older will develop AF [21]. The prevalence of Atrial Fibrillation is 0.1% in younger than 55 years and 3.8% in 60 years or above and 10% in 80 years or older [22]. Atrial fibrillation incidence significance is higher in men than women [23]. Atrial fibrillation is common in white race than in black race. However atrial fibrillation is often associated with other cardiovascular diseases, only 10-15% cases of atrial fibrillation occur in the absence of comorbidities. The risk of stroke from atrial fibrillation is estimated to be 1.5% for the age group of 50-59 years and it approaches 30% for the age group of 80-90 years [24].

Atrial fibrillation can cause auricular fibrillation by forming blood clots that can traverse to brain from the heart, resulting in stroke. Often it start as short period of abnormal beatings which become longer and stays constant for over time [25]. Often episodes may not have symptoms [26].

Sometimes atrial fibrillation may be with an occurance of palpitations, faint, lightheadedness, breatlessness, or chest pain [27]. The disease has an increased risk of heart failure, dementia and stroke [26]. A history of stroke as well as high blood pressure, diabetes, heart failure, or rheumatic fever may indicate whether someone with AF is at a higher risk of complications [28].

In Atrial Fibrillation, the SA node generates a normal regular electrical impulses generated in the right atrium of the heart and it is excited by disorganized electrical impulses usually originates in the pulmonary veins root. This causes irregular conduction of ventricular impulses which createss the heartbeat [29].

The P wave activity can be observed as "coarse fibrillatory" and it is termed as "coarse atrial fibrillation" although there is no clinical significance.

The atrioventricular node intermittently becomes refractory and allows only a certain atrial action potentials to reach the ventricles. This is the cause where the ventricular rate is not also in between 400 to 600 bpm, but rather around 100 to 200 bpm. The degree of action potential which crosses the AV node to the ventricles is variable and AV blocking medications can decrease the action potential.

As due to AV node is intermittently (not regularly) refractory, when an action potential does reach the ventricles the QRS complexes are produced and will occur an "irregularly irregular" manner as there is no pattern to their frequency. This is usually manifests as varying RR intervals.

Diagnostic investigation of AF requires a complete history and physical examination, transthoracic echocardiogram, ECG, CBC, and serum TSH level [29].

Figure No-02: ECG of Atrial Fibrillation

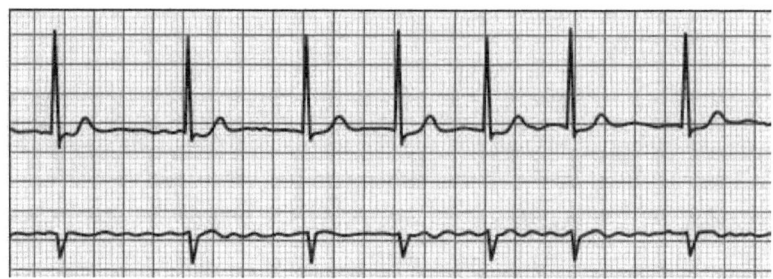

[Image adapted from https://www.quora.com/in/How-do-you-detect-atrial-fibrillation]

In an ECG graph from the Figure no-1 Atrial Fibrillation is understood with Leads V4 and V5. It shows irregular intervals between heartbeats. There are two rhythms that are irregularly irregular are atrial flutter with variable conduction and multifocal atrial tachycardia. Atrial flutter has the typical "sawtooth pattern" whereas multifocal atria tachycardia requires three distinct P wave morphologies in one 12 lead ECG tracing. There are quite few arrhythmias they are regularly irregular, such as 2nd-degree AV block type I (Wenkebach). This indicates atrial fibrillation will be with no P wave and an irregularly irregular QRS complex.

Atrial Flutter:

Atrial flutter can be described as rapid (270 to 330 atrial beats/ min) but regular activation of atria. The ventricular response usually has a regular pattern and a pulse of 300 beats/ min. This arrhythmia occurs less frequently than atrial fibrillation but has similar precipitating factors, consequences, and drug therapy [19].

Atrial flutter is less common than atrial fibrillation. In a study of atrial flutter 75% are men. In patients of atrial flutter with atrial fibrillation older adults tend to be more affective for an average group of 64 years. Incidence of atrial flutter is estimated to be 200,000 new cases per year. The prevalence of atrial fibrillation increases with age from the age group of 25-90 years.

Symptoms of atrial fibrillation can be a feeling of heart beating too fast, too hard, or skipping beats, chest discomfort, difficulty breathing, or loss of consciousness. It typically reflects the decreased cardiac output. Typical symptoms include palpitations, fatigue, mild dyspnea, presyncope and less common symptoms are angina, severe angina or severe syncope. In physical examination pulse may be regular or slightly irregular, possible hypotension. Some other examinations like palpations over the neck and thyroid gland and jugular venous distension, auscultation over the lungs for crackles and heart for extra heart sounds and murmurs and lower extremities for edema or impaired perfusion.

Although this abnormal heart rhythm typically occurs in individuals with cardiovascular disease (e.g. high blood pressure, coronary artery disease, and cardiomyopathy) and Diabetes Mellitus, it may occur spontaneously in people with otherwise normal hearts. Typically it is not a stable rhythm and degenerates oftenly into atrial fibrillation [30].

13

Figure No- 03: ECG of Atrial Flutter

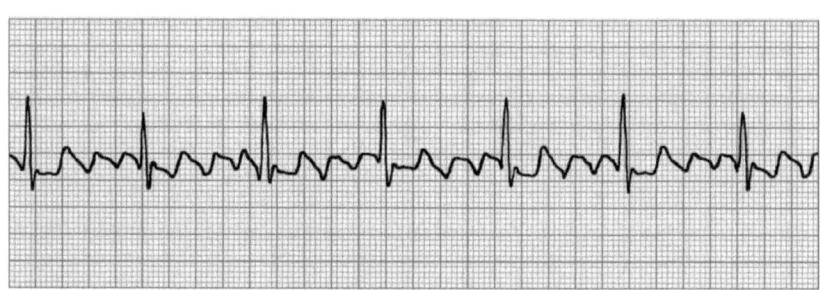

[Image adapted from https://thephysiologist.org/study-materials/atrial-flutter/]

In an ECG graph from the figure no-02 atrial flutter is understood with leads II, III and aVF. Atrial flutter shows variable conduction of the P waves in the ECG graph. There may be a presence three P waves to one QRS complex, then quick change to two P waves to one QRS complex can occur.

Based on anatomic location from where it originates Atrial Flutter can be described as type I (typical) and type II (atypical). It can be discussed as "clock wise" or "counterclockwise" given in figure no-3. It depends on the direction of the circuit.

From a reentrant circuit around the tricuspid valve annulus and through the cavo-tricuspid isthmus, typical atrial flutter rotates counterclockwise in direction. This results in negatively-directed flutter waves in the inferior leads.

From the same reentrant circuit around the tricuspid valve annulus and through the tricuspid isthmus, the direction of circuit can reverse and cause clockwise arial flutter. This results in positively directed flutter waves in the inferior leads.

Diagnosis can be done with the techniques of ECG, Vagal maneuvers, and adenosine administration by blocking AV node, exercise testing, holter monitor.

Atypical atrial flutter originates from the left atrium or in the areas of right atrium, such as surgical scars, and has a variable appearance on ECG in regards to the flutter waves.

Figure No- 04: ECG of counterclockwise flutter and clockwise flutter

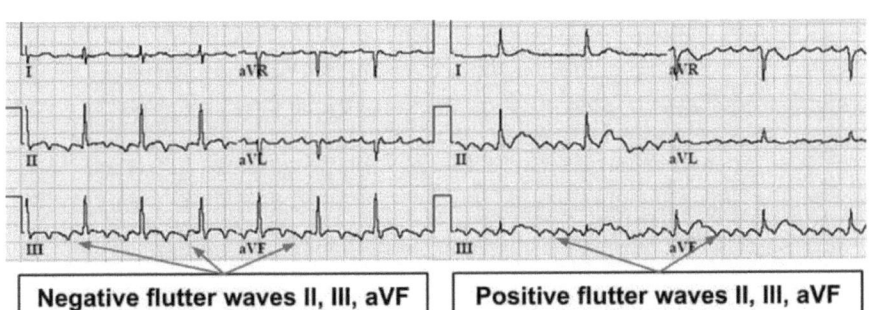

| Negative flutter waves II, III, aVF | Positive flutter waves II, III, aVF |
| Counterclockwise flutter | Clockwise flutter |

[Image adapted from https://www.healio.com/cardiology/learn-the-heart/ecg-review/ecg-topic-reviews-and-criteria/atrial-flutter-review]

Paroxysmal Supra Ventricular Tachycardia:

Paroxysmal SVT is a type of supraventricular tachycardia occurs in an episodic condition with an abrupt onset and termination. Often people have no symptoms. Otherwise symptoms may include palpitations, dizziness, feeling lightheaded, sweating, shortness of breath, and chest pain, diaphoresis and nausea. Episodes start and end suddenly [32].

Paroxysmal SVT is triggered by a reentry mechanism in which it may be induced by premature atrial or ventricular ectopic beats. In adolescents usually have SVT from an accessory pathway [33]. The cause of paroxysmal SVT is not known but some triggering factors include alcohol, caffeine, nicotine, psychological stress, hyperthyroidism, stimulants and Wolff- Parkinson- Whitesyndrome which often is inherited from a person's parents.

Paroxysmal SVT is observed not only in healty individuals but also more common in patients with previous history of mitral valve prolapse, rheumatic heart disease, pericarditis, pneumonia, chronic lung disease, alcoholic intoxication [34, 35]. Toxicity of digoxin has been associated with paroxysmal SVT [36, 37 & 38]. Rare complications of paroxysmal SVT are CHF, MI, sudden drop in blood pressure, and sudden death. Paroxysmal SVT patients with Wolff- Parkinson-White syndrome may have a greater risk for cardiac arrest if they lead to develop atrial fibrillation or atrial flutter in the presence of a faster conducting accessory pathway.

The incidence of paroxysmal SVT is approximate to about 1-3 cases per 1000 persons, with a prevalence of 0.2%. Prevalence of paroxysmal SVT increases with age usually seen in middle aged and older patients.

Diagnosis can be done with an electrocardiogram (ECG) which reveals narrow QRS complexes and a rapid heart rhythm between 150 and 240 beats per minute [39]. An enzyme evaluation for cardiac patient should be done for chestpain and patient with risk factors of myocardial infarction. Other laboratory tests include electrolyte levels, complete blood picture count, thyroid studies and digoxin levels. A chest radiograph suggested for the presence of pulmonary edema and cardiomegaly, a transthoracic echocardiogram for structural or congenital heart disease and Cardiac magnetic resonance imaging (MRI) can be useful to asses congenital heart disease is being considered.

Figure No- 05: ECG of Paroxysmal Supraventricular Tachycardia

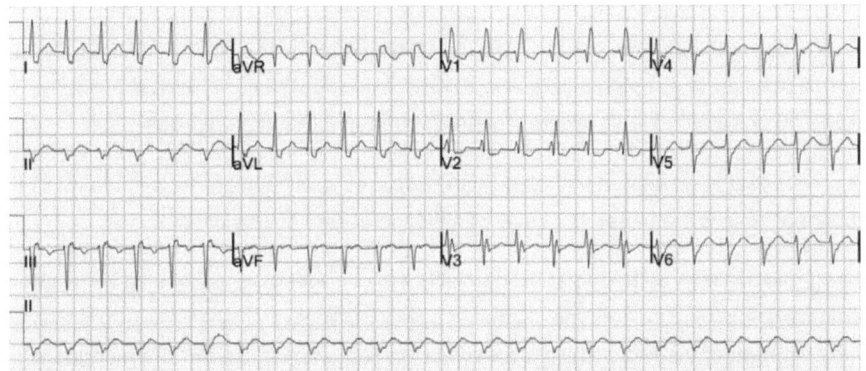

[Image adapted from http://hqmeded-ecg.blogspot.in/2014/01/paroxysmal-svt-psvt-that-repeatedly.html]

In an ECG graph from the figure no-3 of Paroxysmal SVT is understood with the leads of aVR, V1, V4 at zone I, aVL, V2, V5 at zone II and aVF, V3, V6 at zone III. Here rate change occurs in a single beat, rate may increase upto 100-250 beats per minute but most often between 140-250 beats per minute. P waves may not be discernible during the Paroxysmal SVT phase. P- R intervals will be normal if P waves are discernible. There will be narrow QRS complex usually seen in Paroxysmal SVT. Rhythm appears in regularly regular.

Vagal maneuvers, such as the Valsalva maneuver, are often used as the initial treatment. If not effective and the person has a normal blood pressure the medication adenosine may be tried. If adenosine is not effective a calcium channel blockers or beta blocker may be used. Otherwise synchronized cardioversion is the treatment [40].

If the person is hemodynamically unstable or other treatments have not been effective, synchronized electrical cardioversionmay be used for restoring sinus rythm. In children this is often done with a dose of 0.5 to 1 J/Kg [41].

Wolf Parkinson White Syndrome:

WPW is a disorder due to a specific type of problem with the electrical system of the heart which has resulted in symptoms [42]. About 40% of people with the electrical problem never develop symptoms [43]. WPW occurs more commonly in males than females.

A rapid heartbeat is present at birth due to an extra electrical pathway. In patients with WPW an abnormal gene is the cause in a small percentage of people with WPW.

Ebstein's anomaly is a heart defect during child birth considered as congenital heart disease in which the septal and posterior leaflets of tricuspid valve are displaced towards the apex of the right ventricle of the heart which is shown in the figure no-5. The WPW syndrome is also associated with congenital heart disease like ebstein anomaly.

Figure No-06: Difference between normal heart and Ebstein's anomaly

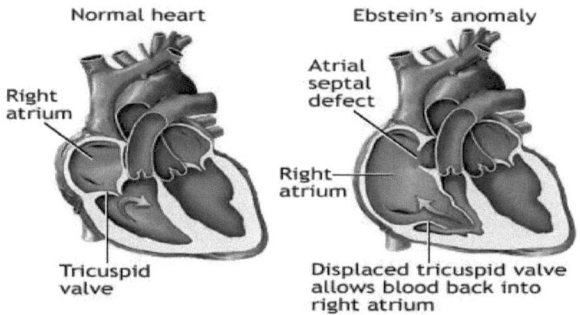

[Image adapted from https://healthjade.com/ebstein-anomaly/]

Patients with Wolff-Parkinson-White syndrome have a bypass tract or an accessory pathway that connects the atria electrical system directly to the ventricles, thereby allowing conduction to avoid passing through the AV node.

In healthy individuals, when the sinus node generates an action potential it must pass through the AV node and to the ventricles. When an accessory pathway is present, the sinus node action potential can pass through the bypass tract before the AV node, which causes the ventricles to become depolarized quickly. This is termed "pre-excitation" and results in a shortened PR interval on the ECG.

Symptoms can include an abnormally fast heartbeat, palpitations, and shortness of breath, lightheadedness, or syncope. Rarely cardiac arrest may occur. The most common type of irregular heartbeat that occurs is known as paroxysmal supraventricular tachycardia [44].

People with WPW are usually asymptomatic when not having a fast heart rate. Individuals may suffer from palpitations, dizziness, breathlessness, or infrequent syncope (fainting or near fainting) during episodes of SVT. Sometimes ECG may reveal the telltale "delta wave".

Especially during during the time of having AV blocking agents, the patients with WPW and potentially atrial fibrillation can be fatal. They have an erratic action potential occurs at 400-600beatsper minute. This action potential can conduct through the accessory pathway very rapidly than through the AV node. Therefore, patients with WPW and atrial fibrillation have greater ventricular rates than those patients without WPW.

Figure No-07: ECG of Wolff Parkinsin White Syndrome

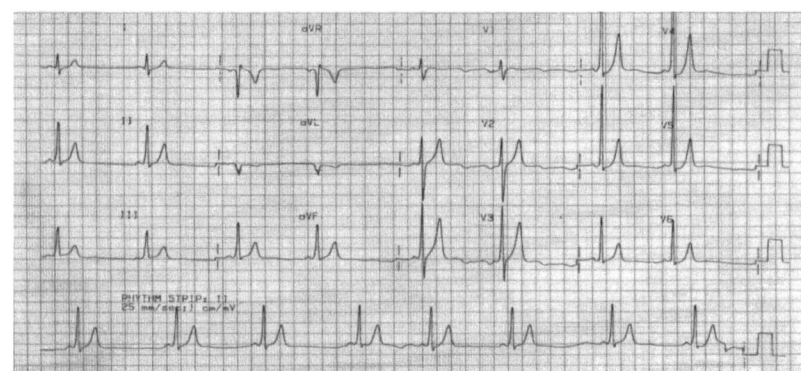

[Image adapted from https://lifeinthefastlane.com/ecg-library/pre-excitation-syndromes/]

Atrio Ventricular Nodal Re-Entrant Tachycardia:

AVNRT is a type of abnormal fast heart rhythm. It is a type of supraventricular tachycardia (SVT), meaning that it originates from a location within the heart above the bundle of his. AV nodal reentrant tachycardia is the most common regular supraventricular tachycardia. The presence of dual AV nodal pathways is the substrate for AVNRT [45].

It is more common in women than men (approximately 75% of cases occur in females). It occurs in young, healthy patients but also in those with chronic heart disease.

There are two pathways which connect into the AV node in AVNR patients. Antegrade conduction occurs over the slow pathways in most of the AVNRT patients, and retrograde conduction occurs over the rapid pathway during AVNRT [46].

When an atria premature complex is blocked in the rapid pathway, an initiation of tachycardia occurs in most of the AVNRT patients but it can conduct via the slow pathway. Although AVNRT patients may have a dual pathway physiology, the fast pathway must have a longer refractory period antegrade than the slow conducting pathway.

Sudden development of rapid and regular palpitations is the main symptom of AVNRT. Often, no provoking factor is identified, although some people affected by AVNRT report developing symptoms in stressful situations, and after consumption of alcohol or caffeine. An abrupt onset and termination is typically characterized in AVNRT. Episodes of AVNRT last from seconds to minutes to days. It is well tolerated in the absence of structural heart disease. Some symptoms like Palpitations, chest discomfort, pounding neck, Nervousness, Anxiety, dizziness [47], shortness of breath, frequent urination can occur after termination of an episode.

Figure No- 08: Conduction Pathway in Normal and AVNRT

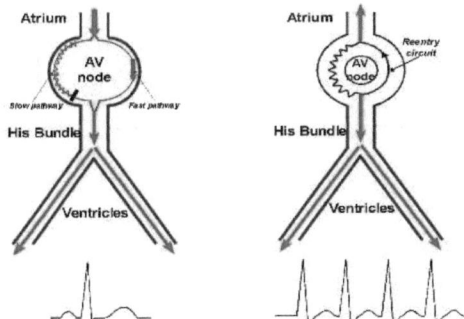

[Image adapted from http://www.washingtonhra.com/arrhythmias/av-nodal-reentrant-tachycardia-avnrt.php]

In patients with coronary artery disease AVNRT may leads to angina or myocardial infarction and still worsen the heart in patients with poor left ventricular function.

A sudden drop in heart rate and blood pressure may occur in patients prolonged tachycardia or a rapid ventricular rate because of poor ventricular filling, decreased cardiac output, hypotension and reduced cerebral perfusion. A decrease in heart rate and blood pressure may occur due to transient asystole when the tachycardia terminates and also due to tachycardia induced depression of the sinus node.

The onset of the fast heart is associated with syncope in some cases. When this occurs, the patient may experience faint. If the heart rate is very fast, and the patient has underlying coronary artery disease (obstruction of the arteries of the heart by atherosclerosis), chest pain similar to anginamay be experienced; this pain is band- or pressure-like around the chest and often radiates to the left arm and angle of the left jaw. AVNRT is rarely life-threatening.

Figure No- 09: ECG of Normal and AVNRT

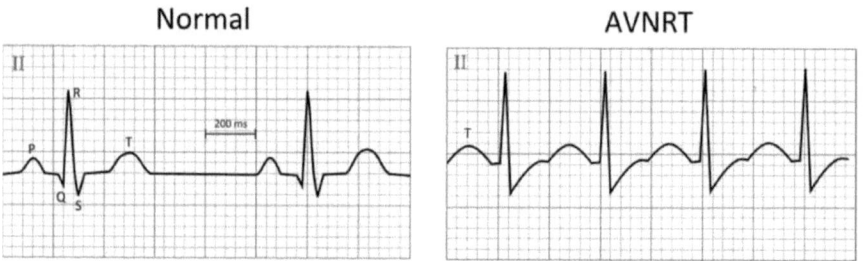

[Image adapted from http://www.nataliescasebook.com/tag/atrioventricular-nodal-reentrant-tachycardia]

An ECG graph from figure no-06 of AVNRT can be termed "dual AV nodal physiology", one pathway is slower and has a short refractory period while the other is faster and has a long refractory period. Normal conduction occurs through the faster pathway with the long refractory period. ECG findings have a narrow complex tachycardia, after the QRS complex formation there will be an immediate P wave occurance indicates as a short RP interval. Tachycardia that can rapidly terminated with AV blocking maneuvers (carotid massage or adenosine).

If a premature atrial contraction (PAC) or less commonly premature ventricular contraction (PVC) occurs at the right time, there will be still a refractory with a normal conduction pathway, thus through the fast AV nodal patway action potential will conduct with the shorter refractory period instead. After reaching this action potential over ventricles or atrium, it will conduct back trough the normal AV nodal conduction patway, as it will be no longer be refractory and a reentrant circuit will be created.

Figure No- 10: Initiation of AVNRT with a Paroxysmal Ventricular Contraction

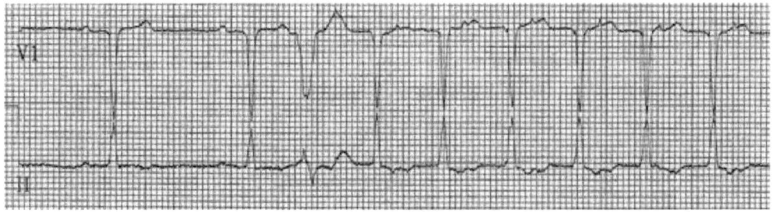

[Image adapted from

https://www.google.com/search?q=initiation+of+AVNRT+with+a+paroxysmal+ventricular+contraction

&source=lnms&tbm=isch&sa=X&ved=0ahUKEwjN9surzOvaAhXLs48KHfxoDnAQ_AUICigB&biw=1

366&bih=613#imgrc=iVJ_K61d1qmMjM:]

Treatment can be suggested initially with specific physical maneuvers, medications, or sometimes synchronized cardioversion. Radiofrequency ablation may require in the condition of frequent attacks, in which the abnormal conducting tissue in the heart may destroy.

Atrio Ventricular Re-Entrant Tachycardia:

AVRT is an abnormal fast heart rhythm and is classified as a type of supraventricular tachycardia (SVT). In patients of AVRT, its common association with Wolff-Parkinson-White syndrome, electrical signals allows via an accessory pathway to enter the atria from the heart's ventricles and cause earlier than normal contraction, which leads to repeated stimulation of the atrioventricular node [48].

The SVT episodes may present with palpitations, dizziness, shortness of breath, or losing consciousness (fainting). In between the episodes of tachycardia the affected person is likely to be with no symptoms; however, the ECG reveals the classic delta wave in Wolff–Parkinson– White syndrome [49].

There are two different pathways involved in AVRT. One is the normal atrioventicular conduction system and other is an accessory pathway. An electrical signal normally passes from the AV node into the ventricles during AVRT, and then the electrical impulse passes pathologically via an accessory pathway into the atria. This causes an atrial contraction and returns to the AV node to complete the reentrant circuit. After its first initiation the cycle may repeats causing the heart to bea faster than usual. AVRT initiation may be through a atrial premature impulse, juntional or at origin of ventricular [50].

When there is a renentrant circuit is present outside of the AV node an atrioventricular reentrant tachycardia occurs through an abnormal conduction pathways that connects to the ventricles from an atrium. This pathway is known as accessory pathway or a bypass tract. In wolff parksinson white syndrome there can be an observation of congenital abnormal accessory pathway.

If an electrical signal is able to travel across the accessory pathway and then returns retrograde through an AV node or vice versa- a reentrant circuit can be created resulting in AVRT.

Figure No-11: ECG of AV

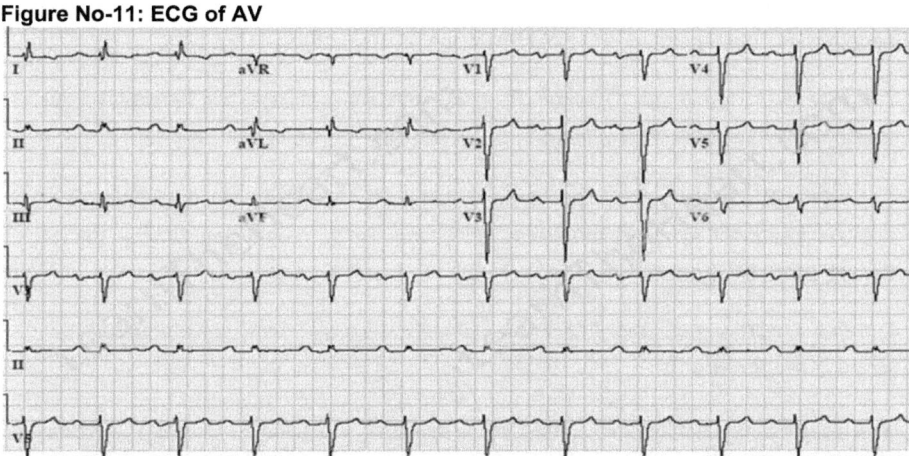

[Image adapted from https://www.healio.com/cardiology/learn-the-heart/ecg-review/ecg-archive/first-degree-av-block-ecg-5]

An ECG graph from figure no-7 of AVRT understood with an observation of a narrow complex tachycardia of SVT and a variable finding depending on the direction of the circuit and location of the accessory conduction pathway.

Treatment of AVRT is general. Interruption of circuit is of important process of treatment. The patients with shock DC cardioversion may be applicable and in the absence of shock AV node electrical signals is needed. This can be done by a trial of specific physical maneuvers like breath holding. If it not effective IV administration of adenosine works by blockade of complete electrical signals at the AV node and interrupts the reentrant electrical circuit. Beta blocker therapy can suggest for long term management and radiofrequency ablation procedures which interrupts an electrical signal via an accessory pathway is also a useful management.

BIBLIOGRAPHY

1. Colucci RA, Silver MJ, Shubrook J. Common types of supraventricular tachycardia: diagnosis and management. Am FAM Physician. 2010; 82(8):942-952.

2. Porter MJ, Morton JB, Denman R, et al. Influence of age and gender on the mechanism of supraventricular tachycardia. Heart Rhythm. 2004; 1(4):393-396.

3. Seslar SP, Garrison MM, Larison C, Salerno JC. A multi-institutional analysis of inpatient treatment for supraventricular tachycardia in newborns and infants. Pediatr Cardiol. 2013; 34 (2):408-414.

4. Gowd BM, Thompson PD. Effect of female sex on cardiac arrhythmias. Cardiol Rev. 2012; 20 (6):297-303.

5. Rosano GM, Leonardo F, Sarrel PM, Beale CM, De Luca F, Collins P. Cyclical variation in paroxysmal supraventricular tachycardia in women. Lancet.1996; 347 (9004):786-788.

6. Daniel sohinki, Owen A Obel et al Current trends in Supra Ventricular Tachycardia management.

7. Xie B, Thakur RK, Shah CP, Hoon VK. Clinical differentiation of narrow QRS complex tachycardias. Emerg Med Clin North Am. 1998 May. 16(2):295-330.

8. Klein GJ, Bashore TM, Sellers TD, Pritchett EL, Smith WM, Gallagher JJ. Ventricular fibrillation in the Wolff-Parkinson-White syndrome. N Engl J Med. 1979 Nov 15. 301(20):1080-5.

9. Josephson ME, Zimetbaum PJ, Buxton AE, Marchlinski FE. Tachyarrhythmias. Harrison TR, Resnik WR, Isselbacher KJ, et al, eds. Harrison's Principles of Internal Medicine New York, NY: McGraw-Hill; 2001.

10. Kantoch, Michal J. "Supraventricular tachycardia in children." Indian Journal of Pediatrics 72.7 (2005): 609-619.

11. Gugneja, Monika, et al. "Paroxysmal Supraventricular Tachycardia." Medscape. Updated: Apr05, 2017.

12. Crawford MH. Supraventricular tachycardias. In: Current Diagnosis & Treatment: Cardiology. 4th edition. New York, N.Y.: The McGraw-Hill Companies; 2014.

13. Neumar RW, Otto CW, Link MS, et al. Part 8: adult advanced cardiovascular life support: 2010 American Heart Association Guidelines for Cardiopulmonary Resuscitation and Emergency Cardiovascular Care Circulation. 2010; 122:S729-S767.

14. Blomström-Lundqvist C, Scheinman MM, Aliot EM, et al. ACC/AHA/ ESC guidelines for the management of patients with supraventricular arrhythmias—executive summary: a report of the American College of Cardiology/American Heart Association Task Force on Practice Guidelines and the European Society of Cardiology Committee for Practice Guidelines, Circulation. 2003; 108(15):1871-1909.

15. Smith GD, et al. Effectiveness of the Valsalva Manoeuvre for reversion of supraventricular tachycardia. Cochrane Database of Systematic Reviews. Sept. 28, 2016.

16. Gerstenfeld, EP, et al. Atrial fibrillation ablation: Indications, emerging techniques, and follow-up. Progress in Cardiovascular Diseases. 2015; 58:202.

17. Olgin JE, Zipes DP (2012). Specific arrhythmias: Diagnosis and treatment. In RO Bonow etal., eds., Braunwald's Heart Disease: A Textbook of Cardiovascular Medicine, 9th ed., vol. 1, pp. 771-824.

18. Page RL, et al. 2015 ACC/AHA/HRS guideline for the management of adult patients with supraventricular tachycardia: Executive summary. Heart Rhythm. 2016;13:92

19. Wells, Barbara G. DiPiro, Joseph T. Schwinghammer, Terry L. Hamilton, Cindy Pharmacotherapy Handbook, 6th Edition, chapter 6.

20. Ferrari R, Bertini M, Blomstrom-Lundqvist C, et al. An update on atrial fibrillation in 2014: from pathophysiology to treatment. Int J Cardiol. 2016;203:22-29.

21. Lloyd-Jones DM, Wang TJ, Leip EP, et al. Lifetime risk for development of atrial fibrillation: the Framingham Heart Study. Circulation. 2004;110 (9):1042-1046.

22. Abdel Latif A, Messinger-Rapport BJ. Should nursing home residents with atrial fibrillation be anticoagulated?. Cleve Clin J Med. 2004;71 (1):40- 44.

23. Alonso A, Lopez FL, Matsushita K, et al. Chronic kidney disease is associated with the incidence of atrial fibrillation: the Atherosclerosis Risk in Communities (ARIC) study. Circulation. 2011;123(25):2946-2953.

24. Avgil Tsadok M, Jackevicius CA, et al. Sex differences in stroke risk among older patients with recently diagnosed atrial fibrillation. JAMA. 2012;307(18):1952-1958.

25. Zoni-Berisso, M; Lercari, F; Carazza, T; Domenicucci, S (2014). "Epidemiology of atrial fibrillation: European perspective". Clinical epidemiology. 6: 213–20.

26. Munger, TM; Wu, LQ; Shen, WK (January 2014). "Atrial fibrillation". Journal of biomedical research. 28 (1)

27. Gray, David (2010). Chamberlain's Symptoms and Signs in Clinical Medicine: An Introduction to Medical Diagnosis (13th edition). London: Hodder Arnold.

28. Fuster, Valentin. Guidelines for the Management of Patients with Atrial Fibrillation: a report of the American College of Cardiology/American Heart Association Task Force on Practice Guidelines and the European Society of Cardiology Committee for Practice Guidelines: Developed in collaboration with the European Heart Rhythm Association and the Heart Rhythm Society. Circulation. 2006;114 (7):257-354.

29. Gutierrez C, Blanchard DG (January 2011). Atrial Fibrillation: Diagnosis and Treatment. Am FAM Physician. 83 (1): 61–68.

30. Bun SS, Latcu DG, Marchlinski F Saoudi N. Atrial flutter: more than just one of a kind. European Heart Journal. 2015;36 (35): 2356-2363.

31. Neumar, RW; Shuster, M; Callaway, CW et al. American Heart Association Guidelines Update for Cardiopulmonary Resuscitation and Emergency Cardiovascular Care. Circulation. 2015;132: 315-367.

32. Ferri, Fred F. (2012). Ferri's Clinical Advisor 2013,5 Books in 1, Expert Consult - Online and Print,1: Ferri's Clinical Advisor 2013. Elsevier Health Sciences. p. 807.

33. Orejarena LA, Vidaillet H Jr, DeStefano F, et al. Paroxysmal supraventricular tachycardia in the general population. J Am Coll Cardiol. 1998;31(1):150-157.

34. Klein GJ, Bashore TM, Sellers TD et al. Ventricular fibrillation in the Wolff-ParkinsonWhite syndrome. N Engl J Med.1979;301(20):1080-1085.

35. Montoya PT, Brugada P, Smeets J, et al. Ventricular fibrillation in the Wolff-ParkinsonWhite syndrome. Eur Heart J. 1991;12(2):144-150.

36. Ganz LI, Friedman PL. Supraventricular tachycardia. N Engl J Med. 199;332(3):162-173.

37. Xie B, Thakur RK, Shah CP et al. Clinical differentiation of narrow QRS complex tachycardias. Emerg Med Clin North Am.1998;16(2):295-330.

38. Josephson ME, Zimetbaum PJ, Buxton AE, Marchlinski FE. Tachyarrhythmias. Harrison TR, Resnik WR, Isselbacher KJ, et al, eds. Harrison's Principles of Internal Medicine, New York, NY: McGraw-Hill; 2001.

39. Al-Zaiti SS, Magdic KS. Paroxysmal Supraventricular Tachycardia: Pathophysiology, Diagnosis and Management. Critical care nursing clinics of North America. 2016;28(3):309–316.

40. Neumar RW, Shuster M, Callaway CW. American Heart Association Guidelines Update for Cardiopulmonary Resuscitation and Emergency Cardiovascular Care. Circulation. 2015;132: 315–367.

41. de Caen AR, Berg MD, Chameides L et al. Pediatric Advanced Life Support: American Heart Association Guidelines Update for Cardiopulmonary Resuscitation and Emergency Cardiovascular Care. Circulation. 2015;132:526–542.

42. WPW, rarediseases.info.nih.gov. 31 December 2012. from the original on 21 April 2017. 30 April 2017.

43. Kim, SS; Knight, BP (May 2017). "Long term risk of Wolff-Parkinson- White pattern and syndrome". Trends in cardiovascular medicine. 27(4): 260–268.

44. Genetics Home (March 2017). "Wolff-Parkinson-White syndrome". Genetics Home Reference. Archived from the original on 27 April 2017. Retrieved 30 April 2017.

45. Braunwald E, ed. Heart Disease: A Textbook of Cardiovascular Medicine. 7th ed. Philadelphia, Pa: WB Saunders; 2004.

46. Janse MJ, Anderson RH, McGuire MA, Ho SY. "AV nodal" reentry: Part I: "AV nodal" reentry revisited. J Cardiovasc Electrophysiol. 1993 Oct. 4(5):561-572.

47. Gursoy S, Steurer G, Brugada J, et al. Brief report: the hemodynamic mechanism of pounding in the neck in atrioventricular nodal reentrant tachycardia. N Engl J Med. 1992;327(11):772-774.

48. Josephson ME. Preexcitation syndromes. In: Clinical Cardiac Electrophysiology, 4th, Lippincott Williams & Wilkins, Philadelphia 2008. p.339.

49. Hampton J. The ECG Made Easy. Elsevier 2008

50. UpToDate: Atrioventricular reentrant tachycardia (AVRT) associated with an accessory pathway.

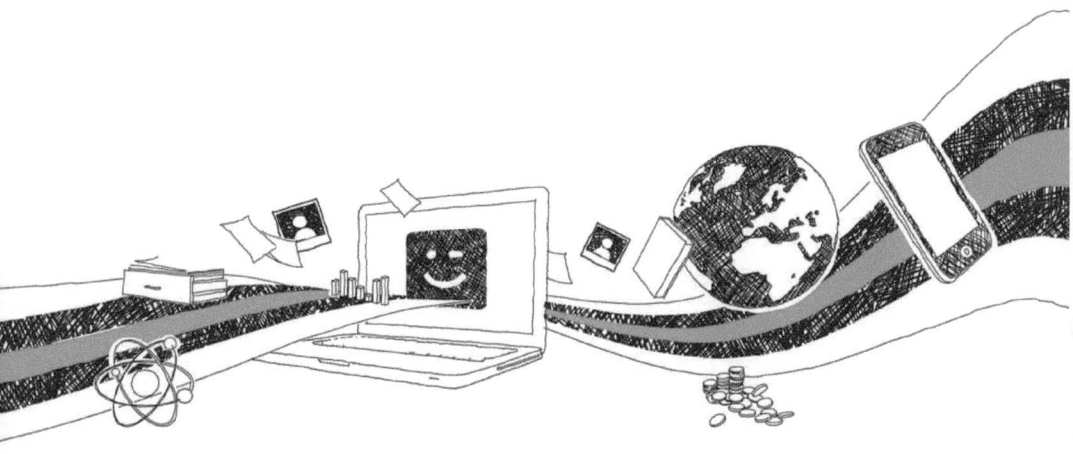
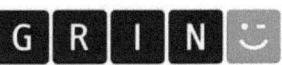